GUIDE FOUR:
SMART PRODUCTS, REAL RESULTS

From Root to Tip: A Growing Hands Guide for Natural Hair

BY CONSTANCE HUNTER

For permissions, inquiries, or additional resources, please contact:

Pre'Vail Natural Hair Salon

www.prevailyournatural.com | prevailyournatural@gmail.com

This book is intended for informational and educational purposes only and should serve as a general guide to understanding and improving natural hair health. While the methods and recommendations provided are based on expertise in natural hair care and trichology, they are not intended to replace professional medical or dermatological advice.

If you are experiencing severe scalp conditions, excessive hair loss, or other persistent issues, it is strongly recommended that you consult a licensed dermatologist or a professional cosmetologist specializing in scalp and hair health. A trained professional can assess underlying causes and provide personalized treatment plans tailored to your specific needs.

By using the information in this book, the reader acknowledges that the author and publisher are not responsible for individual outcomes. Readers should exercise their own discretion when applying the suggested practices.

First Edition: 2025

ISBN:

Paperback: 978-1-968134-04-4

Ebook: 978-1-968134-13-6

Printed in USA

ABOUT THE AUTHOR

As a certified trichologist and natural hair care educator, I specialize in helping individuals discover what's truly possible for their hair—especially when they've been told otherwise.

My passion lies in witnessing transformation—that moment when someone realizes their hair can be healthy, strong, and free. With a deep understanding of the science behind hair and scalp health, I strive to provide clarity, comfort, and actionable solutions. My training equips me to assess and guide care for a wide range of concerns, from common challenges like dandruff and dryness to complex conditions such as alopecia areata, scalp psoriasis, and CCCA.

But my work goes beyond diagnosis or technique. I believe in education, empowerment, and helping clients build routines that nourish their crown from root to tip. This includes learning to read labels, choosing products with purpose, avoiding harmful styling practices, and embracing care that fits their lifestyle and values.

While I offer expert insight from the field of trichology, I'm not a medical doctor. Hair and scalp symptoms can sometimes signal deeper health issues. That's why I encourage a holistic approach—and, when necessary, consulting licensed healthcare professionals for comprehensive support.

In this series, you'll find guidance rooted in science, experience, and care. My hope is that it not only helps you understand your hair better but also love it more, trust it more, and grow with it in ways you never thought possible.

Your hair is not the problem—you just needed the right guide.

DEDICATION

For the one who's bought it all, tried it all, and still feels lost:

It's not you—it's the noise. Let's simplify and start fresh.

OVERVIEW

You don't need a hundred products—you need the right ones. *Smart Products, Real Results* teaches you how to shop with intention, understand ingredients, and choose (or even create) what your hair truly needs. It's time to stop guessing and start selecting with confidence.

No more wasted money. No more one-size-fits-all promises. This guide helps you build a toolkit that delivers real results for your real texture.

SERIES INTRODUCTION

Welcome to *From Root to Tip: A Growing Hands Guide for Natural Hair*

This series was created with one goal in mind: to give you what's been missing—not just products, not just trends, but truth, support, and real guidance for real people who are ready to finally understand and care for their natural hair from the inside out.

For years, we've been taught to manage, fix, or fight our hair. But here, we're doing something different. We're returning to care—not control. To confidence. To consistency. To choice.

Each guide in this series is built as a step in your journey. They can be read in order or on their own, depending on where you are in your process. Whether you're just starting out, rebuilding your relationship with your hair, or deepening your understanding, this space is for you.

I've written these guides from my hands—growing hands that have touched, healed, protected, and restored countless crowns. Now, I offer that care to you.

This isn't just about hair. It's about healing. It's about reclaiming your rhythm, your confidence, and your beauty—from root to tip.

Let's begin.

WHAT YOU WILL LEARN

- How to read and understand product labels and ingredients
- What to look for—and what to avoid—based on your specific hair needs
- How to build a personalized product lineup (cleansers, conditioners, stylers, etc.)
- Common marketing myths and how to spot empty claims
- An introduction to DIY hair care: simple, safe, and effective recipes
- How to balance store-bought products with homemade treatments

WHAT YOU'LL WALK AWAY WITH

- Clarity on what your hair truly responds to
- A simplified, effective product collection (not an overcrowded shelf)
- The ability to shop and mix with purpose—not pressure
- Confidence in your routine and consistency in your results

TABLE OF CONTENTS

INTRODUCTION

Your hair isn't difficult—it's just misunderstood. And often, so are the products we're sold.

In *Smart Products, Real Results*, we break down the science of smart product selection: what's in the bottle, why it matters, and how to make informed choices that support your hair's health and goals. You'll learn to decode labels, avoid common pitfalls, and even explore safe DIY treatments for hydration, strength, and scalp care.

This guide puts the power back in your hands—so your hair can thrive on your terms.

LESSON 1:
CHOOSING THE RIGHT HAIR PRODUCTS

Selecting the right hair products is essential for achieving and maintaining healthy, vibrant hair. The effectiveness of these products largely depends on understanding product labels and ingredients, as well as choosing formulations tailored to your specific hair needs and goals. In this lesson, we'll explore how to navigate product labels, recognize beneficial ingredients, and select products that align with your hair type and objectives.

Understanding Product Labels and Ingredients

Navigating product labels and ingredients can be overwhelming, given the wide range of hair care products available. However, understanding these labels is crucial for making informed decisions. Here's a guide to decoding product labels and identifying key ingredients.

1. Ingredient Lists

Ingredients are listed in descending order of concentration, so the first few ingredients are the most prevalent in the product. Pay close attention to the first five ingredients, as they significantly influence the product's performance.

- **Water (Aqua):** Water is the primary ingredient in most hair products, acting as a solvent for other ingredients. It's essential for hydration and helps distribute the other ingredients evenly through the hair.

- **Cleansing Agents:** Ingredients like sodium lauryl sulfate (SLS) and sodium laureth sulfate (SLES) are commonly found in shampoos because of their ability to create lather and remove impurities. However, sulfates can be harsh on the hair and scalp, especially for sensitive skin or color-treated hair. If you prefer a milder option, look for sulfate-free cleansers like disodium laureth sulfate or sodium coco-sulfate.

- **Conditioning Agents:** Ingredients like silicones (e.g., dimethicone) and conditioning agents (e.g., behentrimonium chloride) provide smoothness and shine. While silicones offer temporary smoothness, they can build up over time, requiring the use of clarifying shampoos to remove. If you prefer to avoid silicones, consider products with natural oils or butters as alternatives.

- **Humectants:** Humectants like glycerin and aloe vera attract moisture to the hair. These are particularly helpful in moisturizing and hydrating hair.

- **Proteins:** Hydrolyzed proteins (e.g., hydrolyzed silk, keratin) help strengthen the hair by filling in gaps in its structure. They are especially beneficial for damaged or weakened hair but can be drying if overused. Products rich in coconut or honey can also provide protein benefits.

- **Preservatives:** Preservatives like parabens and phenoxyethanol prevent microbial growth and extend a product's shelf life. While parabens have been scrutinized for potential health concerns, many products now use paraben-free alternatives.

2. Common Additives and Their Functions

- Essential Oils: Ingredients such as lavender oil, tea tree oil, and peppermint oil offer therapeutic benefits and pleasant fragrances. These oils may have antimicrobial properties and support scalp health.

- Colorants and Fragrances: Artificial colorants and fragrances can trigger allergic reactions or sensitivities in some individuals. If you have sensitive skin, opt for products labeled as fragrance-free or hypoallergenic.

- Thickeners and Emulsifiers: Ingredients like acetyl alcohol and xanthan gum help stabilize and thicken formulations. While they don't typically impact hair health, they contribute to the product's texture and usability.

Selecting Products Tailored to Specific Hair Needs and Goals

Choosing the right products involves aligning your selection with your hair's specific needs and personal goals. Here's a detailed approach to selecting products based on common hair types and concerns.

1. Identifying Your Hair Type

Understanding your hair type is the first step in selecting appropriate products. Hair types are typically categorized by texture, porosity, and density.

- **Texture:** Hair texture ranges from straight to wavy, curly, or coily. Each texture requires different levels of moisture, hold, and styling.

- **Straight Hair:** Typically requires lighter products that won't weigh it down. Look for lightweight shampoos and conditioners that add body without excess oil. A great shampoo and conditioner duo is Sebastian Dark Oil.

- **Wavy Hair:** Benefits from products that enhance waves without causing frizz. Consider curl- enhancing creams or mousses that define waves and add bounce.

- **Curly Hair:** Needs hydrating and curl-defining products to manage frizz and maintain curl shape. Use curl creams, gels, and leave-in conditioners specifically designed for curly hair.

- **Coil Hair:** Often requires intensive moisture and definition. Opt for rich creams, oils, and styling gels that provide hold and hydration.

2. Addressing Hair Concerns

Different hair concerns require targeted solutions, and selecting products that address these issues can significantly improve hair health.

- **Dryness:** For dry hair, choose hydrating shampoos and conditioners with moisturizing ingredients like shea butter, argan oil, and glycerin. Deep conditioning treatments and leave-in conditioners are also beneficial.

- **Frizz:** To combat frizz, use smoothing shampoos and conditioners with silicone alternatives or anti-frizz agents. Look for products that offer humidity control and smoothing benefits.

- **Damage:** For damaged hair, select products with moisture-rich ingredients. Protein treatments, strengthening shampoos, and restorative conditioners can further damage hair if moisture isn't already present — as lack of moisture is often the root cause of damage in the first place. Misuse of products is a common contributor to hair damage.

- **Color-Treated Hair:** Color-treated hair requires products formulated specifically to preserve color and prevent fading. Use color-safe shampoos and conditioners that are sulfate-free and rich in antioxidants.

3. Setting Hair Goals

Align your product choices with your hair goals, whether that's achieving defined curls, adding volume, or maintaining overall hair health.

- **Volume:** For added volume, choose volumizing shampoos and conditioners that lift from the roots. Mousse and rollers can also help enhance body and fullness.

- **Shine:** To boost shine, look for products containing light oils or silicones that create a glossy finish. Shiny hair serums and glossing sprays can provide a reflective shine.

- **Growth:** If promoting hair growth is your goal, consider products with ingredients like lavender oil, rosemary oil, and jojoba oil, which stimulate the scalp and strengthen hair follicles.

4. Reading Labels and Researching Products

Before purchasing, take time to research products and read labels carefully to ensure they meet your needs. Look for reviews from users with similar hair types or concerns to gauge the product's effectiveness. Brands often provide detailed ingredient lists and explanations on their websites, which can help you make informed decisions. Remember, lack of moisture is often the primary cause of breakage, so ensure your products provide adequate hydration.

5. Testing and Adjusting

Hair care is not a one-size-fits-all solution. It may take some trial and error to find the perfect combination of products for your hair. Start with sample sizes or travel-sized products to test new formulations before committing to full-sized bottles. Pay attention to how your hair responds to different products, and adjust your routine as needed. Depending on your hair's condition, it may take 3 to 4 months to break through the barrier and effectively penetrate the hair shaft with moisture.

6. Professional Advice

Consulting with a professional stylist or trichologist can provide personalized recommendations based on your hair type and concerns. Professionals can offer insights into product selection and help you develop a tailored hair care regimen.

By understanding product labels, recognizing beneficial ingredients, and selecting products that cater to your specific hair needs and goals, you can effectively manage and enhance your hair's health and appearance. This approach not only ensures you're using products that work best for your hair but also helps you achieve your desired results with confidence.

LESSON 2:
NATURAL INGREDIENTS AND DIY HAIR CARE

The allure of natural ingredients in hair care lies in their ability to provide gentle yet effective solutions for various hair needs. With a growing interest in DIY hair treatments, learning how to incorporate these ingredients can elevate your hair care routine while offering a creative and personalized approach. This lesson explores the benefits of natural ingredients, highlights commonly used ones in DIY hair care, and provides practical recipes and methods for creating your own products.

Exploring Natural Ingredients for DIY Hair Treatments

Natural ingredients are celebrated for their ability to nourish and rejuvenate hair without the potential drawbacks of synthetic additives. Here's a closer look at some of the most beneficial natural ingredients and their roles in hair care:

1. Aloe Vera

Aloe Vera is well-known for its soothing and hydrating properties. Rich in vitamins A, C, and E, it promotes hair health by reducing dandruff, alleviating scalp irritation, and providing moisture. Its enzymes help clear dead skin cells from the scalp, promoting a healthy environment for hair growth.

2. Coconut Oil

Coconut oil is often praised for its deep conditioning benefits. However, I don't recommend it for everyone. While it's rich in fatty acids that can penetrate the hair shaft, it can block out moisture when used excessively, leading to dry, damaged, and breakage-prone hair. If used incorrectly, coconut oil can be a major cause of dry or damaged hair.

3. Honey

Honey is a natural humectant, which means it attracts and retains moisture. While its moisturizing and conditioning properties may seem ideal for dry hair, it's important to note that, like coconut oil, honey's molecules are small enough to penetrate the hair shaft, potentially blocking moisture and contributing to dry, damaged, and breakage-prone hair. Despite this, honey also has antimicrobial properties that help maintain a healthy scalp environment.

4. Avocado

Avocado is packed with vitamins, minerals, and healthy fats that nourish and strengthen hair. It's rich in vitamins A, D, and E, as well as biotin, which promotes healthy hair growth and repair. Avocado is an excellent choice for deep conditioning treatments, leaving hair soft, hydrated, and revitalized.

5. Olive Oil

Olive oil is rich in antioxidants and essential fatty acids, making it a powerful moisturizer and conditioner. It strengthens hair, reduces breakage, and adds shine. Additionally, it's effective in improving scalp health by alleviating dryness and flakiness, making it a great choice for those with dry or flaky scalps.

6. Jojoba Oil

Jojoba oil closely resembles the natural oils produced by the scalp, making it a great option for balancing oil production. It moisturizes and conditions hair while helping to regulate sebum production, especially useful for those with oily scalps and dry ends.

7. Apple Cider Vinegar

Apple cider vinegar is known for its clarifying properties. It helps balance the scalp's pH, remove product buildup, and enhance shine. However, I would advise using ACV no more than twice a year, as it can be quite drying. If you choose to use it, ensure your hair is heavily moisturized afterward. Personally, I have not used apple cider vinegar in my routine, and many who do report having dry, dull hair as a result.

Recipes and Methods for Creating Homemade Hair Care Products

Creating DIY hair care products allows you to customize treatments to your specific needs. Below are some simple and effective recipes to incorporate natural ingredients into your hair care routine.

Softening Avocado Oil Hair Mask

Ingredients:

- 2 tablespoons of avocado oil
- 1 tablespoon of olive oil
- 1 tablespoon of shea butter

Instructions:

1. Melt the shea butter if it's solidified.
2. In a bowl, mix the melted shea butter with avocado oil and olive oil.
3. Apply the mixture to damp hair, focusing on the ends.
4. Cover your hair with a shower cap and leave the mask on for 30 minutes to an hour.
5. Rinse thoroughly with lukewarm water and style as usual.

Benefits: This mask deeply moisturizes hair, restoring softness and shine. The combination of avocado oil, olive oil, and shea butter nourishes hair, promoting stronger strands and reducing breakage. It's especially beneficial for dry or damaged hair, improving elasticity and hydration without weighing it down.

Gentle Clarifying Rinse

Ingredients:

- 1 tablespoon of apple cider vinegar
- 1 cup of water
- 1 tablespoon of chamomile tea (optional for soothing)

Instructions:

1. Mix the apple cider vinegar and water in a spray bottle or bowl.
2. After shampooing, pour the mixture over your hair or spray it evenly.
3. Gently massage it into your scalp and hair, then leave it on for a few minutes.
4. Rinse thoroughly with cool water.

Benefits: This gentle rinse helps remove product buildup, balances scalp pH, and enhances shine. Chamomile tea can provide additional soothing and calming effects.

Simple Deep Conditioning Mask

Ingredients:

- 2 tablespoons of yogurt
- 1 tablespoon of castor oil
- 1 tablespoon of almond oil

Instructions:

1. Mix the yogurt, castor oil, and almond oil until well combined.
2. Apply the mixture to damp hair, focusing on the ends.
3. Leave it on for 30 minutes, then rinse thoroughly with lukewarm water and shampoo as usual.

   Benefits: This mask hydrates, strengthens, and promotes shine, making it ideal for dry or dull hair.

Aloe Vera and Jojoba Oil Scalp Treatment

Ingredients:

- 2 tablespoons of aloe Vera gel
- 1 tablespoon of jojoba oil
- 5 drops of essential oil (e.g., tea tree or lavender, optional)

Instructions:

1. Combine aloe Vera gel and jojoba oil in a small bowl. Add essential oil if desired.
2. Apply the mixture directly to your scalp using your fingertips.
3. Massage gently for a few minutes to stimulate circulation.
4. Leave the treatment on for 20-30 minutes, then rinse with lukewarm water and shampoo.

   Benefits: This treatment soothes and hydrates the scalp while balancing oil production. It helps alleviate dryness and flakiness, promoting a healthier scalp environment.

Flaxseed Moisturizing Hair Spray

Ingredients:

- 1 tablespoon of flaxseed gel
- 1 cup of water
- 1 teaspoon of jojoba oil

Instructions:

1. Mix the flaxseed gel, water, and jojoba oil in a spray bottle.
2. Shake well and spray lightly onto damp or dry hair, focusing on the ends.
3. Leave it in without rinsing for added moisture and shine.

Benefits: Flaxseed gel provides lightweight hold and moisture, while jojoba oil locks in hydration without greasiness. This spray adds shine, reduces frizz, and promotes healthy, soft hair.

Hair Loss Treatment Oil

Ingredients:

- 2 tablespoons of jojoba oil
- 5 drops of lavender essential oil
- 5 drops of rosemary essential oil

Instructions:

1. In a small glass bottle, combine the jojoba oil, lavender essential oil, and rosemary essential oil.
2. Close the bottle and shake gently to mix the oils.
3. Apply a few drops to your scalp and massage gently for a few minutes, focusing on areas of hair loss.
4. Leave it on for at least 30 minutes, or overnight for best results. Wash your hair as usual.

Benefits: Jojoba oil nourishes and moisturizes the scalp, while lavender oil promotes relaxation and may help reduce hair loss. Rosemary oil stimulates hair growth and improves circulation in the scalp, making this blend beneficial for overall hair health.

Practical Tips for Successful DIY Hair Care

- **Patch Test:** Always perform a patch test before applying any new DIY product to your hair or scalp to ensure you don't have an allergic reaction.

- **Fresh Ingredients:** For the best results, use fresh ingredients. Homemade products should be used immediately or stored in the refrigerator for a short period to maintain their effectiveness.

- **Clean Tools:** Ensure that all mixing bowls, utensils, and application tools are clean to prevent contamination.

- **Adjust Recipes:** Feel free to adjust ingredient quantities based on your hair's length and thickness. For example, longer hair may require more of the mixture.

- **Consistency:** For optimal results, incorporate DIY treatments into your regular hair care routine, but avoid overuse. Balancing them with other products and methods ensures that your hair receives a variety of benefits.

By exploring natural ingredients and creating your own hair care products, you can enjoy customized treatments tailored to your unique hair needs. These DIY approaches not only allow for a more personalized regimen but also promote a deeper understanding and appreciation of the natural elements that contribute to healthy, beautiful hair.

LESSON 3:
READING AND UNDERSTANDING PRODUCT LABELS

Understanding product labels is essential for selecting hair care products that meet your needs while avoiding potential allergens or harmful ingredients. This lesson will guide you through the process of deciphering product labels, enabling you to make informed choices for your hair care routine.

Deciphering Product Labels for Effective Product Selection

Product labels provide valuable information, but they can be overwhelming due to their complexity. To make the most of this information, consider the following key aspects of product labels:

1. Ingredient List

The ingredient list on a product label is typically arranged in descending order of concentration, with the highest concentration ingredients listed first. Understanding this list can help you determine whether a product contains beneficial ingredients or is overloaded with potentially harmful components, such as coconut derivatives.

- **Active Ingredients:** These are the components that provide the primary benefits of the product, such as moisturizing agents, proteins, or vitamins. For example, if you're looking for a hydrating shampoo, check for active ingredients like glycerin, hyaluronic acid, or natural oils. Note that strengthening products often contain a high amount of protein, which can be damaging depending on the health of your hair.

- **Base Ingredients:** These often include water or oils, which serve as the foundation for the product. Base ingredients are essential for the formulation's texture and effectiveness.

- **Preservatives and Stabilizers:** These ingredients extend the shelf life of the product. Common preservatives like parabens or phenoxyethanol can be controversial, so understanding their purpose and potential concerns is important.

2. Ingredient Names

Familiarize yourself with common ingredient names and their functions. Some key categories include:

- **Humectants:** Ingredients like glycerin and hyaluronic acid attract moisture to the hair and help retain it.

- **Emollients:** Oils and butters, such as avocado oil or shea butter, soften and smooth the hair, improving its texture.

- **Surfactants:** These cleansing agents, found in shampoos and conditioners, such as disodium lauryl sulfate or cocamidopropyl betaine, help remove dirt and oil from the hair.

3. Product Claims

Manufacturers often make claims about their products, such as "sulfate-free," "organic," or "for color-treated hair." While these claims can be helpful, they are not always regulated or standardized. Cross-reference these claims with the ingredient list to ensure they align with your hair care needs.

4. Expiry Date and Batch Number

Check the expiry date or batch number to ensure the product is still effective and safe to use. Using expired products can reduce their effectiveness and may cause adverse reactions.

Identifying Potential Allergens or Harmful Ingredients

Being aware of potential allergens or harmful ingredients is essential to avoid adverse reactions and maintain healthy hair. Here's how to identify and avoid problematic components:

1. Common Allergens

- **Fragrances:** Synthetic fragrances can cause allergic reactions or sensitivities in some individuals. If you have sensitive skin or allergies, look for products labeled as "fragrance-free" or "unscented."

- **Preservatives:** Ingredients like parabens, formaldehyde, or formaldehyde-releasing agents can cause irritation or allergic reactions. Opt for products with natural preservatives or those labeled as "paraben-free."

2. Harmful Ingredients to Avoid

- **Sulfates:** Sodium lauryl sulfate (SLS) and sodium Lauretha sulfate (SLES) are common surfactants that can strip natural oils from the hair and scalp, leading to dryness and irritation. If you have sensitive skin or dry hair, look for sulfate-free alternatives.

- **Silicones:** While silicones can provide a smooth and shiny finish, they can build up on the hair over time, leading to dullness and difficulty achieving moisture balance. Consider products without silicones or those labeled as "silicone-free."

- **Alcohols:** Certain alcohols, such as isopropyl alcohol or ethanol, can be drying to the hair and scalp. However, not all alcohols are harmful; fatty alcohols like cetyl alcohol or stearyl alcohol are used as moisturizers and emollients.

3. PH Balance

The pH of a hair care product affects its interaction with the hair and scalp. Products that are too acidic or too alkaline can disrupt the natural pH balance, potentially leading to dryness or irritation. Look for products with a pH balanced to match the natural pH of the scalp and hair (around 5.5). The hair has a positive charge, so conditioners with a negative charge provide moisture and help retain it in the hair.

4. Allergic Reactions and Sensitivities

If you have known allergies or sensitivities, consult the ingredient list for potential triggers. Conduct a patch test by applying a small amount of the product to a discreet area of your skin to check for any adverse reactions before using it on your hair.

Practical Tips for Reading Product Labels

1. **Educate Yourself:** Take time to learn about common ingredients and their effects on hair. The more familiar you are with ingredient names and their functions, the easier it will be to make informed choices.

2. **Use Resources:** Utilize online databases and resources to research ingredients and their safety profiles. Websites like the Environmental Working Group's Skin Deep database provide information on ingredient safety and potential concerns.

3. **Consult Professionals:** If you have specific hair concerns or conditions, consider consulting a dermatologist or a trichologist (a specialist in hair and scalp health) for personalized recommendations.

4. **Test New Products:** When trying a new product, start with a small amount and observe how your hair and

scalp react. Gradually introduce new products to your routine to minimize the risk of adverse reactions.

5. **Keep a Journal:** Maintain a hair care journal to track which products work best for you and any reactions you experience. This can help you refine your product choices and build a routine that suits your hair needs.

Understanding and interpreting product labels empowers you to make better decisions about the products you use on your hair. By paying attention to ingredient lists, avoiding potential allergens and harmful components, and aligning product choices with your specific hair needs, you can achieve healthier, more vibrant hair while avoiding unnecessary complications.

QUIZ:
HAIR PRODUCTS AND INGREDIENTS

Lesson 1: Choosing the Right Hair Products

1. Question

What is the primary reason for reading product labels before purchasing hair care products?

a) To find the most expensive option.

b) To understand the ingredients and their effects on your hair.

c) To select products with the most artificial ingredients.

d) To check how the packaging looks.

Answer: b) To understand the ingredients and their effects on your hair.

INFORMATION NOT COVERED IN LESSON

2. Question

What should you avoid when selecting products for sensitive scalps?

a) Products with natural oils.

b) Products containing sulfates and parabens.

c) Products with water as the first ingredient.

d) Products enriched with vitamins and minerals.

Answer: b) Products containing sulfates and parabens.

Lesson 2: Natural Ingredients and DIY Hair Care

1. Question

Which natural ingredient is commonly used to moisturize dry hair, but may be more damaging than helpful?

a) Coconut oil.

b) Baking soda.

c) Lemon juice.

d) Alcohol-based products.

Answer: a) Coconut oil.

2. Question

What is a key benefit of creating DIY hair care products?

a) You can avoid natural ingredients.

b) You control the ingredients and avoid harmful chemicals.

c) It guarantees better results than store-bought products.

d) It takes less time than using commercial products.

Answer: b) You control the ingredients and avoid harmful chemicals.

3. Question

Which of the following is a popular natural ingredient used for scalp treatments in DIY hair care?

a) Aloe vera.

b) Salt water.

c) Vinegar.

d) Sugar scrub.

Answer: a) Aloe vera.

Lesson 3: Reading and Understanding Product Labels

1. Question

When reading product labels, what does it mean if "aqua" or "water" is listed as the first ingredient?

a) The product is primarily oil-based.

b) The product is formulated to provide moisture.

c) The product is not recommended for natural hair.

d) The product contains more water than any other product.

Answer d) the product contains more water than any other product.

2. Question

Which ingredient is often used as a preservative in hair products and can cause sensitivity for some people?

a) Jojoba oil.

b) Parabens.

c) Shea butter.

d) Coconut milk.

Answer: b) Parabens.

INFORMATION NOT COVERED IN LESSON

3. Question

What should you do if a product label lists an ingredient that you are allergic to?

a) Ignore it and proceed to use the product.

b) Perform a patch test before using the product.

c) Use double the amount of product to see its effect.

d) Return or avoid using the product.

Answer: d) Return or avoid using the product.

CLOSING NOTE

You don't need every product on the shelf.
You just need to know what your hair *truly* needs—and
now you do.